MW01230526

THE
Intimate
Couple's
HANDBOOK

Improving your sex life and
improving your marriage go hand in hand.

JIM AND CARRIE GORDON

The Intimate Couple's Handbook

Copyright © 2018 by Jim and Carrie Gordon

Published by Lazarus Media Productions
www.lazarusmediaproductions.com

All rights reserved. No part of this book may be reproduced, stored in a retrieval system, or transmitted in any form or by any means — electronic, mechanical, photocopying, recording or otherwise — without prior permission in writing from the publisher. The only exception is brief quotations in critical articles or reviews.

ISBN 978-0-9940592-9-1

Contact Us

To book Jim and Carrie to speak at your
church, event, or conference, or to reach them
with any questions, contact them at:
contact@theintimatecouple.com
or reach out to them via social media:
facebook.com/intimate.couple.

Contents

Part 3: Practical Ways to Increase Intimacy

Part 1

INTRODUCING A DREAM MARRIAGE

CHAPTER ONE

Introduction

MONEY, GLAMOUR, AND mind-blowing sex are the core elements of a perfect marriage! ... according to Hollywood.

We're Jim and Carrie Gordon and most definitely *not* writing from Hollywood. Our life is full of challenges and struggles, and we've had our fair share of grief and disappointments. In spite of that, we enjoy a dream marriage!

We Have Our Dream Marriage— Even though It's Not Perfect

Our marriage, while not without problems, is a relationship of sacrificial love, mutual respect, and covenantal commitment. We do our best to live for each other's well-being and joy. We're proud of one another, we compliment and esteem each other, and we endeavour to meet each other's deepest needs. Sex is frequent and fun!

In our lives as pastors and in the writing and speaking we do through The Intimate Couple website, we work hard at helping others with their marriages. Investing in young couples preparing for a life of marriage ahead of them is a blast! Our investment in others keeps us young and vibrant. Recently an older friend relayed to us a comment from her young adult daughter, "Mom, I can't believe Jim and Carrie—they act like they're still teenagers!"

A Dream Marriage Is Available to Any Couple

"Wait a minute," you say. "You don't know my marriage, my husband/wife, or our problems. I just know I couldn't have the kind of relationship you're talking about."

The truth is, a dream marriage is available for any couple willing to quit the default 'me-centred' way of life, and embrace spouse-first mentality. How do we know this? Well, over the past two decades, we have helped hundreds of couples deepen their intimacy and experience their own dream marriage.

Could it be that your situation is similar to so many others who have experienced great improvement?

In this handbook, we want to give you keys to your dream marriage.

- You'll learn that your dream marriage is a combination of emotional, intellectual, spiritual, and sexual intimacy.

- You'll learn that sexual intimacy is only a part... though an integral one... of your dream marriage.

- You'll learn practical ways to increase all four types of intimacy in your marriage.

First, we'll give you a short self-diagnostic tool to see where some of the issues in your marriage might be.

Next, we'll help you understand the four critical types of intimacy that make up a dream marriage.

Lastly, we'll give you clear, practical, useful tips for addressing some of the issues that may have shown up in the self-diagnostic tool.

Ready to dive in? Here we go!

CHAPTER TWO
Self-Evaluation

LET'S GET STARTED with the self-diagnostic tool.

Check all of the following statements that apply to you:

Your Spiritual Connection

☐ I pray throughout the day for my spouse.

☐ We pray together regularly.

☐ We read/study the Bible together.

☐ I am comfortable sharing with my spouse what God is teaching me.

☐ For Wives Only: my husband actively leads me spiritually.

☐ For Husbands Only: I take my role as spiritual leader of my wife/family seriously.

☐ During times of conflict, we pray together inviting God to help each of us change.

Your Mental (or Intellectual) Connection

☐ I pay attention to my spouse's interests and hobbies.

☐ I feel that my spouse supports me in my personal interests.

☐ We are so busy that we only have time to "connect" at the end of the day.

☐ My spouse and I enjoy discussions that help us learn more about what we believe and think on a lot of topics.

☐ I find I get distracted easily when my spouse is talking with me.

☐ My spouse's choice of interests and hobbies make me feel proud of him/her.

☐ I feel free to express my opinion even though my spouse may disagree with me.

☐ We agree on what our core values and beliefs are.

☐ Because of our commitment to one another, I fully trust my spouse and can be vulnerable with him/her.

☐ My spouse rarely interrupts me when I'm talking.

☐ My spouse spends more time in front of the TV or computer than communicating with me.

Your Romantic (or Emotional) Connection

☐ I feel cherished and cared for by my spouse.

☐ My spouse and I enjoy romancing one another.

☐ We say "I love you" to one another often.

☐ My spouse and I spend quality time together almost every day.

☐ I enjoy spending time in conversation with my spouse.

☐ My spouse is my very best friend!

☐ We have learned how to handle conflict with one another.

☐ We still hold hands in public.

☐ My spouse surprises me with love-letters, small gifts, and other expressions of romance.

☐ For Wives Only: my husband usually remembers special dates (Valentine's Day, my birthday, our anniversary)

☐ For Husbands Only: I rarely forget to celebrate special dates.

☐ My spouse expresses his/her appreciation of me and what I do.

☐ My spouse is still holding a grudge even though I've asked for forgiveness.

☐ We almost never go out for a "date night" or a "weekend getaway" with just the two of us.

Your Sexual Connection

☐ My spouse and I are comfortable talking about sex.

☐ We laugh and have fun during sex.

☐ My spouse and I know where to find the female g-spot.

☐ Our sex life has improved in the past year.

☐ My spouse and I kiss more now than in our first year of marriage.

☐ I initiate sex at least 25% of the time.

☐ We try to include variety in our sexual relationship.

☐ I feel my sexual needs are being met.

☐ I've told my spouse what feels good and what I enjoy in our sexual relationship.

☐ My spouse is not as interested in sex as I am.

☐ I struggle with pornography.

☐ Sometimes I find sex boring.

☐ There are new things I'd like us to try when having sex, but I'm too embarrassed to ask my spouse.

☐ For Wives Only: I rarely experience orgasm.

☐ For Husbands Only: my wife has difficulty reaching orgasm.

☐ We are so busy that sex is usually rushed.

☐ I am often too tired for sex.

☐ Sometimes I don't feel sexually confident with my spouse.

Select the word that best describes your sexual relationship with your spouse:

☐ Non-Existent

☐ Disappointing

☐ Boring

☐ Take it or Leave it

☐ Sub-Standard

☐ Adequate

☐ Improving

☐ Pleasurable

☐ In a Good Place

☐ Almost Perfect

☐ In Heaven!

On average, how often do you and your spouse have sex?

☐ Always: at least once a day

☐ Often: several times per week

☐ Regularly: once per week

☐ Occasionally: 2 or 3 times per month

☐ Seldom: less than once per month

☐ Rarely: "We go without sex for months at a time."

So, how did you do?

Where is your marriage at? Do you see any patterns? Are there any specific areas you need extra help?

If you're like most every other married couple out there, you probably see there's room for growth and improvement. Before skipping ahead to Part 3 where we list practical suggestions for how to develop deeper intimacy, let's take a closer look at what intimacy in a marriage actually is.

CHAPTER THREE

What Does a Dream Marriage Look Like?

In a Dream Marriage,
Needs Are Met

It's important to begin the conversation of meeting needs by stating that ultimately, God is the Source for our marriage. He alone is responsible to meet our needs. That being said, does God use a husband to meet his wife's needs? Absolutely! Does God use a wife to meet her husband's needs? Definitely!

But we are not perfect. Our own effort and strength is insufficient to provide one another with the love, acceptance, and value we crave. In light of this, what can we do? Well, we rely on God. Each day, we confess our inability to perform on our own—and we ask Him to live through us. We ask Him to love our spouse through us.

So, if we are trusting Jesus to work through us, does that mean we stop working at our marriage? Do we stop trying, and give up any effort to meet each other's needs? Of course not! If Jesus is living through us, we should expect to work, because He worked—hard! We work to love one another and meet each other's needs.

And Jesus shows up, giving us the strength, insight, and desire to love each other like Him!

Understanding Carrie's Needs

In our dream marriage, I (Jim) understand that Carrie needs to feel cherished, valued, and honoured. She is looking forward to growing old together with me, and not allowing the busyness of life to crowd out those precious, special moments between us. She also loves the idea of my constant admiration of her poise and beauty—both the internal and external kind of beauty!

Understanding Jim's Needs

In our dream marriage, I (Carrie) have come to understand that Jim connects emotionally with me through sex—and so, sexual intimacy is part of what we need in our marriage! Jim also needs to be respected and honoured. He delights in me being his best cheerleader!

In a Dream Marriage, Joy Is Found

Every healthy marriage relationship has one common ingredient—joy. Joy is not freedom from problems or worry: it is the result of an attitude of thanksgiving, appreciation, and gratitude. This attitude lifts and lightens the heart and makes it joyful!

Loving rituals are those little peculiarities expressed between husband and wife—unique to them—that say, "I love you. You're special!"

The book, *What Happy Couples Do* by Bruess and Kudak, tells one story of a husband and wife who race to be the first to write a secret loving message with a toothpick on the smooth surface of each new jar of peanut butter!

In a Dream Marriage, Forgiveness Is Practiced... Often!

(From Jim) I won't ever forget the time I hurt Carrie through a thoughtless, selfish act. Feeling shame, and overcome by guilt—I asked her to forgive me. I felt broken and vulnerable—believe me, it wasn't pretty! Carrie was so awesome—she was as gracious and forgiving as she could be—making me feel accepted and approved independent of my poor behaviour. How can I not love a wife like that!

You would be amazed how many couples tell us their spouse is holding a grudge (even after they've asked for forgiveness), and they don't feel forgiven about something in their past. We believe that many couples don't actually know HOW to forgive!

They say that time heals all wounds, but that would be wrong. Time heals clean wounds. When you are hurt in a marriage, it's because your spouse, through their actions, has taken something from you. Perhaps it's your sense of value or security. They may have taken your sense of worth or belonging. Regardless, you are left with a deficit. You're left wounded.

Unaddressed and unforgiven, your wound will fester into bitterness and resentment. Forgiveness cleanses the wound—allowing it to heal. Does forgiveness mean you don't feel pain anymore? No, a clean wound still hurts. But now, the pain is a reminder that Jesus is our source—not our spouse. And, as time goes on, the clean wound will heal.

Forgiveness says this:

"I forgive you. Through your actions, you took (my sense of belonging, value, significance, etc.) from me, and I've been longing for you to pay me back and make it up to me somehow. But right now, I forgive you that debt. You don't owe me anymore. How can I say that? Because Jesus has offered to pay the debt you owe me—and I accept His offer. Today, He is the one I look to for validation. He is the one who has filled those deficiencies. He has restored the holes your actions left."

Forgiveness like this truly cleans our wounds, allowing us to heal.

Building a Dream Marriage

We've discussed several aspects of the dream marriage, but the question remains: how can my marriage become my dream marriage? The answer is simple: Strengthen and develop intimacy between you and your spouse.

For more on that, keep reading!

CHAPTER FOUR
The Intimacy Iceberg

WE LIKE TO use the analogy of an iceberg to convey the different forms of intimacy. We have all heard that the tip of the iceberg is only about 10% of the entire structure; what lies beneath the surface of the water is massive compared to what is visible to the eye. The huge mass of ice below the water's surface determines the speed and direction the iceberg flows. In the same manner, what is under the surface of a marriage makes all the difference, in every area.

Over the last few decades, we've worked with many marriages and observed that, when most couples talk about intimacy, they're usually thinking sex. However, the reality is that sex is just the tip of the marital intimacy iceberg. Below the surface lie three other types of intimacy: intellectual, emotional and spiritual.

Let's dig into each of the four types of intimacy.

Intellectual Intimacy

Reflecting on intimacy rarely causes people to consider the mental or intellectual connection as important. Typically, it's romance (the emotional intimacy) and sex (the physical intimacy) that are always centre-stage when we think of intimacy in marriage.

Yet, isn't it true that one of the most powerful agents in binding one person to another is the awareness that "Finally! Here is a person that who really understands me!"

Intellectual intimacy is, in our opinion, the most overlooked of the four intimacies.

We can always detect the clear signs that a couple is having marriage problems, and all marriage problems are really intimacy problems. When we notice that couples dismiss or disregard each other's words, opinions, and thoughts or when a couple is not actively listening and trying to understand one another, intellectual intimacy is gone and the relationship is in jeopardy.

Emotional Intimacy

It is in this particular area of closeness that romance best fits into the picture. When our emotions are involved, things get very interesting! It's all the warm, cozy feelings of falling in love and being in love that we think of when we consider emotional intimacy.

All of the words, thoughts, and actions that affect how we feel about our spouse and about our marriage have a bearing on emotional intimacy.

Spiritual Intimacy

Based on the bedrock of common values and beliefs, spiritual intimacy extends our oneness to the very core of who we are, and influences how we perceive ourselves and the world around us.

Arguably the most neglected type of intimacy, spiritual intimacy is also the most important, because it is a tri-intimacy involving husband, wife, and God. Our relationship with God is like the hub of a wheel. Everything else comes into balance when the Lord has central position in our lives.

In the marriage vows, husband and wife make a vow to each other in the sight of God. Our vows include God and our ability to fulfill those marriage vows is directly linked to how well we trust and rely on Him. As we look to God to love our spouse through us, we find that He does—and our marriage thrives.

Sexual Intimacy

The other three forms of intimacy can be experienced between any two people; however, it is the sexual relationship (reserved between husband and wife) that makes marriage the most unique of all relationships. In a healthy marriage, "sexual intimacy" means that both partners are interested in sex, and their knowledge of their spouse's sexual interests is growing and deepening as well.

Unless you consciously work on deepening the four areas of intimacy, the initial excitement of the relationship, the 'spark', or the "honeymoon stage" will fade away. The realities of life: busyness, tiredness, financial stress, family, and health issues can certainly dampen things. Issues creep in and take priority.

Couples that DO choose to engage with the Intimacy Iceberg will experience their dream marriage—and the benefits are huge!

- passion re-ignited

- deepened intimacy

- relationship with their spouse transformed

- they experience the DREAM MARRIAGE and have better and better sex

In the following pages, we show you exactly how to nurture and develop each area.

Part 2

UNPACKING THE FOUR
TYPES OF INTIMACY

CHAPTER FIVE

Intellectual Intimacy in Marriage

MARIE WAS 25, Stan was 34, and their marriage was in a rocky spot. While they shared belief in the basic tenets of Christianity, there were many issues that Marie had questions about. Stan, however, was completely uninterested in engaging with his wife's honest questions, beyond a trite reply of, "It's true because God said so."

Marie deeply desired a home where open, honest questions were valued. But as Stan consistently shut such conversations down, she began to despair of that every being a possibility. As time went on, Stan's control become more forceful and condescending. He'd belittle Marie's questions, refusing her attempts for open conversation.

Like Stan and Marie, many couples suffer from a lack of intellectual intimacy. They do not realize its importance as a vital component to an overall sense of closeness. In fact, if one partner fails to respect the thoughts and questions of the other, their relationship is heading for disaster.

The mental connection or intellectual intimacy may well be the most overlooked form of intimacy. Yet, it is this closeness that usually first binds two people together. Granted, a man may be attracted by the physical appearance of a woman, but it is the mental connection developed through getting to know each other intellectually that first draws a couple to each other.

Many couples feel that "spark" of excitement growing between them as they spend time conversing and becoming good friends with each other. This process begins intellectually and quickly becomes emotional as well.

It's almost impossible to separate a couple's intellectual relationship from their emotional relationship—they're so tightly woven together, it's almost the same thing! Nevertheless, unless we continue to develop intimacy with our minds and intellect, our relationships become stale—even sex is impacted!

The Four C's Of Intellectual Intimacy

Communication

To experience closeness here requires the ability to convey what you are thinking to your partner as clearly as possible, confident that whatever you say or think will be valued.

Caring

Caring, in this context, is willingness to entertain new thoughts and ideas, and come to a deep level of understanding. Caring results in giving each other the mutual freedom to think independently so one partner does not dominate the other, demanding that they think the same way about everything. It is best defined as being able to be myself—I can be just me, without fear that my thoughts or ideas will be rejected or demeaned.

Commitment

When commitment is present in a relationship, then both husband and wife fully know (mentally) that their spouse is loyal and can be fully trusted. They understand each other.

Common Values

As related to mental closeness, common values represent the same world view, or philosophic approach to life. Both husband and wife are seeing their world through the same lenses.

CHAPTER SIX
Emotional Intimacy in Marriage

AFTER JUNE AND Alfred got married, both put on weight. Several years later, June began exercising and eating healthy. She lost weight. Alfred, though, did not change his lifestyle, and was soon 100 pounds overweight. Shortly after that, Alfred began complaining about his wife's healthy cooking, choosing to eat cakes and greasy food he bought at the corner store. He also began making fun of his wife's body.

June was hurt by this of course, and concerned because of the high risk of Alfred developing diabetes, which ran in his family. Additionally, she no longer found her husband sexually attractive, which brought enormous feelings of guilt and shame.

While the problems plaguing this marriage at first seem to be solely a result of Alfred's overeating, the reality is that there are other, deeper issues. Issues which can't be identified until Alfred is willing to confront his emotional dysfunction. Without individual emotional health, emotional intimacy in marriage is not possible.

A soulmate connection is a phrase that sometimes defines emotional intimacy. It describes a deep bond between a husband and wife. There are those who distinguish between the two phrases by assuming emotional intimacy is developed, whereas a connection between soulmates is automatic—ordained and heaven-sent. Let's assume that a soulmate bond and emotional intimacy are essentially the same thing: then, whether developed or made in heaven, there are four characteristics.

The Four C's of Emotional Intimacy

Communication

When couples are able to accurately convey their feelings to each other without intimidation, worry of reprisal, or embarrassment, they are on their way to relating within a context of acceptance. Let's face it, this often requires learning better conversation skills. Tough? Yes, but the results are well worth it! It's so important for couples to learn how to forgive one another to keep the barriers to communication from preventing intimacy.

Caring

Authentic caring promotes openness, honesty, and vulnerability to know and be known by your spouse. Couples who practice this authentic caring will inevitably also experience a renewed sense of freedom. Imagine feeling free to completely be yourself, with no pretense, regardless of other people's expectations! With this in place, a soulmate bond will naturally lead to understanding each other on a very deep level!

Commitment

There is no better definition of emotional intimacy than a connectedness that exists when two people are enjoying the benefits of commitment and trust toward each other. Each is committed to the well-being and development of the other; each fully trusts the other, and knows they are perfectly safe with one another. It's interesting to know, at this point in a relationship the non-verbal communication is every bit as valuable as the words that are spoken!

Common Values

Holding common, fundamental beliefs and core values results in couples seeing and "feeling" the world in the same way. This mutual emotional perspective is a sure sign of a soulmate connection.

In this type of relationship, couples will begin to discover that any conflict that might arise between them can actually be a tool to bring deeper levels of intimacy!

CHAPTER SEVEN

Spiritual Intimacy in Marriage

SPIRITUAL INTIMACY, WHILE often difficult to attain, is actually the most significant type of intimacy. Why? It powerfully impacts the other three areas. Many couples find it rather awkward to develop. We suspect the reason for this lies in the nature of spiritual intimacy. If you think about it, spiritual intimacy is really a tri-intimacy: closeness among three: husband, wife, and God!

There are a number of critical components or building blocks needed to develop that close spiritual relationship.

The Four C's of Developing Spiritual Intimacy

Communication

Talking about our spiritual journey and experiences with each other...and with the Lord... is the basis of everything here! Prayer is part of the process of increasing that special close relationship. Many couples are hesitant about praying out loud with each other. It is really a matter of practice, realizing we can talk to Jesus like we would another person right beside us!

Caring

Caring for your spouse's spiritual life involves openness, honesty, and vulnerability. Coupled with this caring is a freedom for both husband and wife to be completely themselves, regardless of the perceived expectations of their spouse. Closeness with the Lord and with each other isn't possible if we feel the pressure (internally or externally) to be someone other than ourselves.

Commitment

We need to see both sides of commitment: obviously, it applies to couples being totally committed to each other. At the same time, though, the spiritual dimension of the relationship grows as the husband and wife, together, experience a growing commitment to God, and a trust in Him!

Common Values

Couples don't have to necessarily believe all the same things; nevertheless, unless there are fundamental common beliefs and core values, there can be no spiritual unity. When one partner is Christian and the other is Muslim, for example, there can be no intimacy spiritually.

When a couple prays together on a regular basis, spiritual intimacy between that husband and wife is greatly increased. The habit of praying together is essential and foundational for building a divine connection in couples.

CHAPTER EIGHT
Sexual Intimacy in Marriage

MY HUSBAND AND I have been married for 17 years, together for 20. I have become "sexless" and my husband is bored with just "routine sex". My question is, how can I be more pleasing to him to keep him happy? I just fell into a state of really not wanting to have sex at all. I love my husband, very deeply, but sex is the last thing from on my mind.

He is always looking up ways to please me, and he acts on them. I am very pleased, obviously, and he is left out in the cold. I feel horrible for allowing this to happen! I want us to have a healthy relationship, sexually and mentally. I told him I would try toys, after he asked. He also wants me to masturbate, to learn my body, and I tried, but I was not able to achieve an orgasm.

I feel like I am doing wrong, even though he enjoys the thought, and I was wondering if I should feel wrong, or just enjoy it also? I am willing to do whatever I have to, to make him enjoy me again, because I do enjoy him. What do you recommend?

Rather than record our response to our reader, we have included this question for another purpose: when you read her question, it becomes very apparent that the kinds of problems couples have in their sex lives can be incredibly complex!

We don't want to convey the idea that a simplistic approach will lead everyone to the resolution of all their difficulties. What we can definitively state, though, is that when a couple follows through with the simple principles of intimacy we're talking about, changes can occur that will lead to significant steps forward.

In the case of our reader, focusing on emotional, intellectual, and sexual intimacy is critical. They need to talk about her feelings related to sex, and communicate clearly so they understand each other fully. In addition, we would point them toward learning about respecting an individual's conscience by referring them to our article: "Christian Views on Sex" (visit our website: theintimatecouple.com and search for the article).

Sexual intimacy in marriage is critical to a healthy, happy relationship between husband and wife. Along with the emotional, intellectual, and spiritual aspects, God designed husband and wife to enjoy the experience of sexual intimacy in marriage: intimacy, as we've just defined it, is the ultimate human experience!

Love, marriage, and sex are the three building blocks making sexual intimacy possible. Love—contrary to the vast majority of songs on the radio about this topic—is about meeting the needs of others and is not about self-gratification. Obviously, you don't need marriage to have sex; but you certainly do need marriage to experience the authentic, powerful, and enjoyable sex God intended!

Love, sex, and marriage without the relational emphasis is just the sexual act; it leaves people empty, dissatisfied, and feeling guilty. This explains just one reason why pornography is so destructive (even apart from the terrible psychological addiction): it delivers a momentary, addictive pleasure without the core dimension of intimacy.

The Four C's of Sexual Intimacy in Marriage

Communication

Frustration builds when a husband and/or wife are not able to communicate about problems, desires, fears, or a host of other regularly unspoken issues that impact their sexual experience. Communication allows difficult topics to be openly discussed. What if the wife has no interest in sex? On the other hand, is there freedom to share sexual fantasies with your spouse? Can both partners openly share what they think about their sex life, as well as every other part of their lives?

Caring

Caring for your partner means providing them with the sexual experience that pleases them, on their terms, in their way, in their time frame. A husband caring for his wife might mean he focuses on slow and gentle caresses, speaking of her beauty and his love for her, or perhaps practicing giving a full body massage.

Commitment

Commitment to sexual intimacy in marriage involves doing what is necessary to achieve it, and eliminating whatever is necessary that impedes it. Commitment also translates into time: you must prioritize your time for sex since busyness is one factor that will prevent sex from happening.

Common Values

When couples hold different values, standards, and ideals unity becomes incredibly difficult, if not impossible. Couples holding opinions which are by definition mutually exclusive can never agree—unless one of them changes. For example, if you and your partner have major differences in deeply held religious convictions, then you've hit an impasse.

For sexual intimacy to blossom in a relationship, compatibility is vital. It's not that couples need to agree on everything, but they have to feel safe to hold their own values and ideals without threat or conflict: this is how trust is built. With this trust in place, couples can be honest and open knowing they are accepted and valued.

Part 3

PRACTICAL WAYS TO
INCREASE INTIMACY

CHAPTER NINE
Increasing Intellectual Intimacy

TODD WAS UNTEACHABLE. He refused to see things from his wife, Mala's perspective. On rare occasions, he'd magnanimously give in and allow his wife to have her way; but he pouted and didn't let her forget that he was giving in because he's such a great guy. This attitude was eroding the intimacy in his marriage.

We were able to communicate to Todd the importance of intellectual intimacy. As he applied our techniques and strategies for developing meaningful conversation, he discovered a new sense of unity with Mala—even though the two of them still had their disagreements.

This extreme story perfectly illustrates the fact that without intellectual intimacy, there is no intimacy of any kind. Intellectual intimacy is actually a function of meaningful communication.

And so, meaningful conversation is one of the true cornerstones of every successful relationship, and it deepens intellectual intimacy as well. Asking great questions is an excellent way to improve both intellectual and emotional intimacy.

One of the best places to begin is by asking your spouse thoughtful, conversation-starting questions. These questions will promote:

- active listening

- conversation

- learning to respond better in conflict

- tolerance and understanding

Many of us become lazy and simply stop learning about our "significant other". Invest the time to ask deep, thoughtful questions that develop intellectual intimacy and promote discussion in a safe, accepting setting.

Develop Intellectual Intimacy with Questions

Ask Open-Ended Questions

These are questions that can't be answered with a "Yes" or "No", but require a more thoughtful response. For example, "If you could go back in time and change your career path, what would you change, and why?"

Reminisce About the Positives of Your Past

Be specific about questions. Here's an example: "Honey, I remember you remarking, 'Our vacation to SeaWorld in Florida was our best vacation ever!' What happened to make you feel that way?"

Frame questions about past vacations and trips, family events (birthdays, anniversaries, weddings, etc.), friends and family, satisfaction from employment, hobbies, and community volunteerism. Once you get the hang of it, asking great 'reminiscing' type questions will come easily!

Dream About Your Future Together

Step outside the limitations you feel right now about yourself and, with your spouse, dream about what you hope happens five, ten, fifteen, or twenty years out. Ask questions that help you define what you want that future to be! Describe the details of your answers as vividly as possible:

Where are you going to be living?

What service club could you volunteer with?

List specific hobbies or part-time vocations in which you could invest time.

Top 10 Tips for Increasing Intellectual Intimacy

1. Become a better listener, not just to hear but to understand. Take turns listening to one another's opinions. Ask questions that show you fully understand your spouse's viewpoint.

2. Include your spouse in your personal decision-making. Ask yourself, "Do I demonstrate that I value my spouse's opinion as much as (or even more than) my own?"

3. Do you know what interests and dreams your spouse has?

4. Have you both divulged personal secrets to each other, in an expression of openness and humility?

5. Have a heart-to-heart conversation, asking your spouse: "Are there specific times that I have ridiculed or made fun of your opinion? I need to know because I realize that is very wrong and not honouring to you at all."

6. Ask your spouse: "Do I often dominate our conversations?" Give your spouse freedom to think for themselves.

7. Acceptance of differing opinions is a critical core value. Discuss with your spouse the best ways to value each other's uniqueness. Compose a list, "Ways You and I are Different— but that I Wouldn't Want to Change!"

8. Identify your partner's top two interests. Creatively determine how you can encourage them in those interests.

9. Look for opportunities to compliment your spouse on their thoughtful opinion—privately and publicly.

10. Are you your spouse's best cheerleader? Being a great cheerleader means knowing about the interests and dreams your spouse has. It means valuing their opinion. It means learning them.

CHAPTER TEN

Increasing Emotional Intimacy

*Discover How Marital
Conflict Can Result in a
Stronger Marriage*

To be honest, we've had moments of marriage conflict during our 35 plus years of marriage. Our relationship has had its ups and downs. We've discovered that marriage is a path and a journey… albeit the most wonderful journey of our lives.

Both of us avoid discord and controversy whenever we can. We're uncomfortable in any situation where it is necessary to confront one another or anyone else for that matter. We'd choose to experience a relationship that is always peaceful, full of harmony, and in a state of calm serenity.

...But we have many lessons to learn in life, and it seems God has chosen the marriage relationship to be the classroom for many of those lessons. Could it be that relationship conflict can actually be helpful in changing us to be a better spouse? Could working through the issues that initiate arguments between us actually help to deepen our love for one another?

We've experienced times in our marriage when serious marriage conflict issues brought an emotional separation between us. Any of these issues, unaddressed, had the potential of doing serious damage to our relationship. We remember how one time, as difficult as it was, we faced the challenge and talked about it (both of us in humility and tears). The outcome? ...An expression of our renewed love and commitment to one another, the resolve to not hurt one another again, and a time of praying together thanking God for protecting our marriage.

It was amazing! In the end, the very thing that brought pain also brought us closer than if we hadn't had the conflict. We remember the heightened level of emotional intimacy we felt after working through the conflict. Benefits of working through conflict between a husband and wife may include:

- a "touchpoint" that results in communication

- learning to accept one another's differences

- a recommitment to our relationship

- a renewed appreciation for the value of the love we share

- a rekindled dedication to protect our marriage relationship

- personal growth in character as each spouse learns to respond correctly to the other and chooses to be a better husband or wife

- a greater awareness of our need for God in our relationship

Don't despair when you experience marriage conflicts. Welcome those times with a commitment to properly work through the issues with love and humility. Allow yourself to be vulnerable and uncomfortable (no conflict is ever pleasurable), aware that you and your spouse will reap rewards of a deeper level of intimacy.

Non-Verbal Communication

Communication in relationships may very well be the critical component of success in developing intimacy. Ignorance of your partner's personality, background, style of interaction, and love language all cause communication barriers that will prevent intimacy. When addressing this problem, however, we almost exclusively think of spoken words. Given that "actions speak louder than words", it's easy to understand why non-verbal communication is so important to the development of intimacy. The question remains… how do you build intimacy without words? Here are just a few examples of non-verbal communication:

- Putting your arm around her shoulders

- Gently touching her arm, shoulder, or back whenever you pass each other

- Smiling at one another from across the room

- Linking arms with his

- Holding hands

- Making eye contact with one another in a crowd

- Holding the door open for her

- Caressing her cheek

- Stroking his hair

- And of course, there's always hugging and kissing!

Of all the ways to nurture intimacy, communicating non-verbally is by far the most powerful. A gentle touch or caress bridges the barriers between two lovers. Although surrounded by many people, even the meeting of eyes with a knowing smile can provide a "caress" from a distance!

Let's face it, most men can use improvement in this category! Most women need non-sexual touch to feel cherished, and yet something as simple as touch is often overlooked. Take our list and practice at least a few of the ways to communicate non-verbally every day. The key is consistency. You won't be disappointed with the results!

Top 10 Tips for Increasing Emotional Intimacy

1. Say "I love you" often!

2. Steal time away to connect with your partner, especially when you're busy.

3. Schedule a weekly husband/wife meeting: it's a date night... with purpose! Take time to discuss personal and family goals, as well as goals for your marriage. If you'd like, write down progress in the areas you are working on in your relationship.

4. Many women connect emotionally through words, affection, and non-sexual touching; many men connect emotionally through sex. Discuss together how this applies to you. Include non-sexual touching in your daily interaction with your spouse. Hold hands more often, steal kisses, be playful!

5. Treat your spouse better than you would a guest in your home!

6. Identify any destructive habits you and your spouse have during conflict. Talk about them and establish ground rules. For example: no belittling, no raised voices, no interrupting each other.

7. Agree to speak in lower, softer tones when you are in conflict. Proverbs 15:1 is a great rule to live by!

8. Develop vulnerability by saying how you really feel—as awkward and difficult as it may seem at the moment.

9. Learn to be clear when you forgive one another: acknowledge personal responsibility for the hurt feelings; ask forgiveness clearly. (Don't say "If I hurt you, I'm sorry"..."If?" Of course you hurt them, so acknowledge it and

ask for forgiveness.)

10. Decide to forgive again and again and again!

CHAPTER ELEVEN

Increasing Spiritual Intimacy

Practice Praying Together

We have experienced many wonderful benefits as we've learned to pray together. For one, the practice helps keep our focus where it belongs: Jesus Christ is the centre of our marriage.

Second, God is invited to participate in our lives. His power brings strength and protection to our relationship. Listen to what we can read in the Bible in the Book of Ecclesiastes 4:12. "A cord of three strands is not easily broken." What a blessing we experience when we together, through prayer, agree with God to follow and live in His ways.

Third, we agree to give the concerns we face to God instead of worrying, arguing, or disagreeing about them with one another.

Fourth, our deepest longings and fears are often revealed when we open our hearts to God before one another. This might seem terrifying at first, but what a beautiful thing it is to reveal your fear and have your spouse accept you in spite of that! Not only that, but each of us will come to know best how to pray for one another.

In addition, we've discovered that our love for one another increases as we pray for each other. Our love expands and deepens when we pray for our spouse. It's difficult staying angry or annoyed with someone you're praying for.

If you and your spouse are not practicing this godly habit, please... make the commitment today to spend time daily in prayer together. Praying together is so powerful! You and your spouse are not just two individuals praying but a united couple.

In Matthew's gospel (chapter 18 verse 19) we read how Jesus said, "If two of you agree down here on earth concerning anything you ask for, My Father in heaven will do it for you."

Use these few basic "how to's" to help you and your spouse pray together effectively:

- Find a time and place to pray that is free from distractions.

- Kneel or sit down together.

- Hold hands.

- Take turns praying aloud. If you aren't used to praying in front of others, this is the best way to learn.

- Don't pray too long. (This is not the time to "preach" to your spouse.)

- Pray a blessing for one another.

- Be sure to pray and ask God to help you be the spouse you need to be.

Here are three other suggestions you might like to try when praying with your spouse.

Conversational Prayer

Let's say the husband begins praying out loud for a brief time, then the wife picks up where he leaves off. After a moment, she pauses and the husband prays again. Continue praying back and forth until you are done.

Pray Scriptures Together

Find selections of the Bible to use as prayers. In fact, you may find that many of the Apostle Paul's writings include prayers. Try this with Ephesians 1:16-20 or Philippians 1:9-10.

Pray About Your Concerns

As you and your spouse are in discussion about topics, whether they are to do with your own relationship, your children, family, health, work, or whatever may be of a concern to you, take a moment to stop your discussion and pray about the matter.

Top 10 Tips for Increasing Spiritual Intimacy

1. Make your spiritual life measurable: how do you invest time, money and resources when it comes to your spiritual life?

2. Block out time on the calendar to engage in activities that you mutually agree will enhance your spiritual life together.

3. Describe to your spouse how you would rate your spiritual life on a scale of 1 to 10. On

what basis do you make this evaluation? Discuss with each other your feelings and expectations about spirituality in your relationship.

4. Read the Bible and other spiritual literature together and share your insights.

5. Talk about your past spiritual journey: how was God leading you—first as individuals, and then as a couple?

6. God has given you desires, passions, and gifts! Write them down and ask yourselves: "How are we using our desires, passions and gifts for the Kingdom of God?"

7. Pray together regularly as a couple: hold hands and take turns praying (as you pray and ask, remember also to seek and listen).

8. Commitment grows with trust. Ask your spouse: "Do you see any discrepancies be-tween what I say and how I live that might have eroded some trust between us?"

9. Pray for your spouse throughout the day, and express your gratitude for them often.

10. Encourage your spouse in the truth. Speak truth over them, and remind them how God sees them.

CHAPTER TWELVE

Increasing Sexual Intimacy

WE'LL DIG A lot deeper into sexual intimacy in the next chapters, but here are 10 quick tips for increasing sexual intimacy right away:

1. Men, sex starts in the kitchen. Being helpful in the kitchen, preparing dinner together, or washing the dishes can actually be a turn on for your spouse.

2. Foreplay: take plenty of time... 20 minutes minimum. Husbands, learn to slow down. Try keeping all your clothes on while you engage in foreplay with your wife.

3. Educate yourselves more about sex. Why not attend a seminar, take a course online, read books together, or check out our website? Be sure to look for information for Christian mar-

ried couples.

4. Discuss together why open communication about sex can be difficult. Do both of you feel safe in expressing feelings? Are you able to identify influences that make openness a challenge?

5. Ask your partner what they like, what they would like to try, and what doesn't work for them during sex.

6. Become a student of your spouse, and improve your techniques. There is always room for growth no matter how long you've been married.

7. Discuss and come to agreement on what's okay or acceptable in your sexual relationship, and what you must avoid.

8. Agree together that you will meet each other's intellectual, emotional, spiritual, and sexual needs, and will not allow other people to meet those needs.

9. Together, acknowledge the importance of sex in your relationship. Prioritize time for sexual intimacy—put it in your private calendars, if necessary.

10. As a partner, your goal is to please your spouse; remind your lover that your next love-making session is all about pleasuring them and making them happy.

Guys, This Section Is for You

Men, to experience and share great sex with your wife, be sure to use some of these sexual foreplay tips. There is an art to foreplay. Don't just grab and squeeze, or head straight for her privates. Foreplay IS NOT five minutes of kissing and fondling breasts before intercourse. It's about courting and wooing your wife's sensual responses and arousing her sexually.

Foreplay is part of the preparation phase of love-making.

Foreplay is focusing on helping your wife come to sexual arousal.

Foreplay must not be rushed. Spend at least 20 to 30 minutes on foreplay.

The process starts before you hit the bedroom!

- kiss her gently in public

- touch her face and stroke her hair

- tell her you love her

- hold hands or put your arm around her in public

- tell her she's beautiful

In the bedroom, as things start warming up...

- slowly start undressing her

- give her tender kisses on the lips

- gently stroke her face

- take time to give her a full body or shoulder massage

- gently caress all parts of her body (not just the usual "sexy" parts)

- whisper and tell her how beautiful she is and how good she feels

- kiss her softly all over her body

- interlace your fingers with hers

- caress her tummy ... without tickling!

- touch and fondle her

- keep talking about how much you love her

- try to discover new touch points on her body that are sensitive and bring sexual arousal

- keep looking at her

Foreplay Tips to Use as Things Get Hot

- begin passionate kissing (don't underestimate this tip!)

- start faster stroking and caressing of her body

- include full body embracing

- start oral stimulation such as licking and sucking

- begin to caress her inner thighs

- continue telling her all the ways you think she's gorgeous and how much she excites you

- squeeze and stroke her body

Final Sexual Foreplay Tips

- move your hands from the top of her body all the way down between her legs

- listen to your wife's verbal cues… is she feeling discomfort or pleasure?

- use lubricant to begin stroking her vagina and clitoris

- gently massage her outer vaginal lips

- pay attention to your wife's body language; is she beginning to respond?

- ask your wife to tell you what feels good to her

- reach up to fondle her breasts

- kiss her passionately all over her body

- massage her inner thighs

- stimulate her clitoris and/or g-spot until she lets you know she's ready for intercourse or ready to orgasm

- don't forget to keep talking to her; tell her how much you enjoy her body

Guys, as you use these tips, you'll experience new levels of intimacy in your sexual relationship with your wife including increased awareness of your wife's body and how she responds, and great orgasm experience for both you and her.

So, remember:

1. Start Slowly and Gently

2. Speak Lovingly

3. Don't Rush

4.   Use Lubricant

5.   Pay Attention to How She Responds

Increasing Sexual Desire (From Carrie, for Women)

Typically, I have a lower sex drive and libido. In fact, there are times when I have no interest in sex at all. It may be that I am too busy, distracted, or tired. Still, I understand that my sexual relationship with Jim is so important. Not only does it fulfill a need he has, but it's also an important way that Jim and I connect physically and emotionally.

Because of the importance of sex in our marriage, I will find ways to increase my sexual confidence, knowing that I will boost sexual desire in myself as a result. If you have little or no interest in sex, let me suggest that you begin to use the following suggestions to gain it back.

- You Initiate Sex: Most of us women expect that if our husband wants sex, he will take the lead, but he would be so excited if you initiated sex. And… it's amazing, you'll find that you will gain sexual confidence and desire yourself!

- Prepare Yourself All Day: Playful hugs, lingering kisses, loving phone calls or texts are just a few simple ways to help you prepare yourself ... and your husband ... for a passionate time of sex later in the day.

- Passionate Kissing: Don't pass up the best way to increase passion and sexual desire. Be sure to communicate your love in the very basic but very powerful expression... the kiss. Spend time embracing and passionately kissing.

- Give Enough Time for Sex: Be sure there is plenty of time for foreplay and that you won't feel rushed. Running out of time is a sure way to kill your sexual desire.

- Keep Your Thoughts on Topic. Don't let yourself get distracted by what you need to do (laundry, kids, work...). Whisper loving thoughts to your husband to help keep your mind involved with your love-making.

- Be Aggressive: Rid yourself of inhibitions and be the aggressive sexual partner once in a while. Your husband will probably be aroused by your boldness. Don't keep yourself too relaxed or you may find yourself falling asleep before sex is done.

- Try Something New: A new position, a new

location, new lingerie, a new time of day... Don't let your times of intimacy be predictable or boring. Keep them hot!

- Treat Your Husband: Find out what especially delights him and then do it. Become a student of your spouse and make it your goal to please him out of this world. The best sex is when we want to gratify our spouse more than ourselves.

- Educate Yourself: Visit the bookstore or library or do some online research to find out how to have great sex. (Caution: Avoid the research whose content violates your spouse's and your moral values.) Though there is some value to innocence and self-discovery, sometimes becoming educated will help you learn to overcome barriers to sex or learn how to enhance love-making.

Go for it, ladies! Don't wait for lost interest in sex to come back on its own. Take steps to take it back and increase sexual desire.

CHAPTER THIRTEEN

Increasing Sexual Confidence

SEXUAL CONFIDENCE IS achieved when love, passion, and proficiency work together. This section addresses achieving sexual confidence. It's written by me, Carrie. I hope this will help women become more sexually proficient.

Though I'm still working through my sexual inhibitions, I've learned a greater freedom as I've understood the importance of becoming sexually proficient and having sexual confidence.

"When love and skill work together, expect a masterpiece." — *John Ruskin*

Biology teaches us the "how to have sex." I remember my father giving my sister and I the "where babies come from" biology lesson. In grade 6, my school nurse taught the girls in our class about puberty, and hormones, and body changes. Since being married and giving birth to our nine children, I've read countless articles and books, taken classes, watched movies, compared notes with other expectant or new moms, and asked my doctor questions. I wanted to become more knowledgeable about pregnancy and childbirth.

I've been eager to learn what I needed to know for these "basics". Admittedly, I've also researched, studied, taken courses, and attended seminars regarding health, my occupation, raising a family, homemaking, and hobbies. But why have I been hesitant to teach myself about the area of my sexual relationship with my husband, who is the most important person in my life?

Sex Was God's Idea

I realized I had this preconceived notion that sex was man's idea. But it's not! Do you think God was surprised when He saw Adam and Eve having sex for the first time?

"Stop, guys! What do you think you're doing?"

Of course not! He knew exactly what we would do and designed for sex to happen.

Since God designed us to experience sex, I believe He wants me to do it to the best of my ability. Once I understood the importance of sex, I became motivated to spend time and effort in learning how to please my husband better, be fulfilled in my womanhood, and enjoy sex.

Shame Doesn't Belong

I discovered that we women don't need to feel ashamed for desiring to learn more about sex, how to get better "in bed", and how to become great lovers. It's never too late for a wife to improve her sexual skills. Whether you're just getting ready to be married or have already celebrated many anniversaries, remember that anything worth doing is worth doing well. Important note (not just for women): be sure to look for info on sex that doesn't infringe on your values.

My change in attitude resulted in increased enjoyment and confidence.

Do you know what's been so great about becoming more sexually proficient and gaining more confidence in my sexual relationship with my husband? I find that not only does my husband enjoy the experience so much more, but so do I! I don't just "get through it" but can "relish" sex from beginning to end.

"There is no greater spiritual exchange between a man and a woman than that of lovers loving well."
— *Lou Paget*

CHAPTER FOURTEEN

60 Tips to Deepen Intimacy

Developing Spiritual Intimacy

1. Make your spiritual life measurable: how do you invest time, money, resources on your spiritual life?

2. Pray together regularly as a couple: hold hands and take turns praying about issues, other people, and for each other.

3. Share with your spouse what you believe God is saying to you today.

4. Husbands: lead your family with regular devotions of some kind.

5. God has given you desires, passions, and gifts: write them down and ask yourselves how you

are using them for the Kingdom of God.

6. Talk about your past spiritual journey: how was God leading you—first as individuals and then together?

7. Pray for your spouse throughout the day.

8. Describe to your spouse how you would rate your spiritual life on a scale of 1 to 10. On what basis do you make this evaluation? Discuss with each other your feelings and expectations about spirituality in your relationship.

9. Encourage your spouse with truth about how the Lord sees and accepts them.

10. Commitment grows with trust. Ask your spouse: "Do you see any discrepancies between what I say and how I live that might erode trust between us?"

11. Block out time on the calendar to engage in activities that you mutually agree will enhance your spiritual life together (pray together, read a book together).

12. Take time to write down your views on the Bible, Christianity, and the Lordship of Jesus Christ. Reaffirm your mutual commitment to these values.

Developing Emotional Intimacy

13. Treat your spouse better than an invited guest to your home.

14. Give undivided attention when your spouse is speaking to you.

15. Say, "I love you" often.

16. Steal time away to connect with your partner, especially when you're busy.

17. Include non-sexual touching in your daily interaction with your spouse. Hold hands more often.

18. Many women connect emotionally through words, affection, and non-sexual touching; many men connect emotionally through sex. Discuss together how this applies to you.

19. Decide to forgive again and again and again!

20. Write love letters to help keep romance alive.

21. Men: it's the thought that counts—so think of ways to cherish your wife... and then do them.

22. Read a book together on developing communication skills for speaking and listening.

23. Learn to be clear when you forgive one another: acknowledge personal responsibility for the hurt feelings and ask for forgiveness clearly. (Don't say, "If I hurt you".)

24. Develop vulnerability by saying how you really feel—as awkward and difficult as it may seem at the moment. Work towards total openness and no secrets with your spouse.

25. Agree to speak in lower, softer tones when you are in conflict. Proverbs 15:1 is a great rule to live by.

26. Decide to follow etiquette rules that help foster and demonstrate respect for each other. Husbands—why not choose to always open the car door for your wife?

27. Schedule a weekly husband/wife meeting—a date night. Make a binder and use it to write down progress in the areas you are working on in your relationship. Try these areas: demonstrating respect for each other, romantic exercises, dealing with conflict.

28. Let's consider conflict resolution: what activities do you engage in that are hurtful to your spouse when you are in conflict?

29. Establish agreed-upon ground rules for conflict in the future (and, yes, conflict is inevi-

table). Your values need to be reflected in the tough times!

30. Avoid using the phrases "you never" and "you always" when working through areas of conflict.

Developing Intellectual Intimacy

31. Ask your spouse if you are always dominating conversation.

32. Become a better listener: don't just hear—strive to understand.

33. Include your spouse in your personal decision-making.

34. How do you ensure you're giving freedom to your spouse to think for themselves?

35. Do you know what interests and dreams your spouse has?

36. Be your spouse's best cheerleader!

37. How do you demonstrate that you value your spouse's opinion as much as your own?

38. Choose to discuss a topic where you know you and your partner disagree. Take turns listening to one another's opinion. The goal

is not to prove you are right! The purpose is to ask questions that demonstrate you fully understand your spouse's viewpoint.

39. Look for opportunities to compliment your spouse on their thoughtful opinion—privately and publicly.

40. Have one of those heart-to-heart conversations to ask the following question: "Are there specific times that I have ridiculed or made fun of your opinion? I need to know because I realize that is very wrong, and not honouring to you at all."

41. Identify your partner's top two interests. Creatively determine how you can encourage them in those interests.

42. Acceptance of differing opinions is a critical core value. Discuss with your spouse the best ways you both can value each other's uniqueness.

43. Try composing lists for each other: "Ways You and I are Different—But that I Wouldn't Want to Change!"

Developing Sexual Intimacy

44. Start sex "in the kitchen"! Men, helping your wife with dishes or supper cleanup will help your wife relax and feel positive about you.

45. Foreplay: take plenty of time... 20 minutes minimum.

46. Don't forget to include lots of kissing.

47. Ask your spouse what they would like to try.

48. Prioritize time for sexual intimacy.

49. Relax, have fun and enjoy one another.

50. Become a student of your spouse, and improve your techniques... no matter how long you've been married.

51. Talk together about why open communication about sex is sometimes difficult. Do both of you feel safe in expressing feelings? Are you able to identify influences that make openness a challenge?

52. Ask your partner what they like, and what doesn't work for them during sex.

53. Read a book together about sex, or consult www.theintimatecouple.com. These provide a forum for discussion about sex and your

sexual practices.

54. As a partner, your goal is to please your spouse; remind your lover that your next love-making session is all about pleasuring them and making them happy.

55. Husband, slow down! Try keeping all your clothes on while you engage in foreplay with your wife for 30 minutes.

56. Read *The Act of Marriage* by Tim and Beverly LaHaye to better understand the importance of sex in marriage.

57. Plan to educate yourselves more about sex for married couples. Why not attend a seminar, take a course online, or read books together?

58. Discuss and come to agreement on "what's okay" in your sexual relationship, and what practices you must avoid.

59. Agree together that you will meet each other's intellectual, emotional, spiritual, and sexual needs, and will not allow other people to meet those needs.

60. "Do your homework" to find out what the Bible really says about sex, and come to agreement on the core values of sexuality and obeying God's Word.

CHAPTER FIFTEEN
Conclusion

EVERYTHING IN THIS book is based on the premise that intimacy is the ingredient in marriage that all of us long for—and, truthfully, that few experience to the degree they desire.

It is no surprise when we examine the stats for divorce, sexless marriages, and dissatisfaction in relationships that our generation and the next are in serious trouble. There exists a startling contrast between technical connectivity with social media, and authentic relationships. The loneliest people could easily be super-active on multiple social media platforms, and yet have no real friends.

Developing intimacy takes effort, and requires a good degree of honesty and transparency—both of which can be scary and makes one feel vulnerable.

Yet, this is the very nature of intimacy. This willingness to be open and honest is the prerequisite to intimacy.

Assuming you, the reader, indeed have this desire—this prerequisite—then *The Intimate Couple's Handbook* was designed with you in mind. It was a book of practical ideas, and "how-tos". We can't give you the desire to cultivate intimacy: but we can certainly put into your hands the tools you need to develop the experience everyone wants, but few people enjoy—deep, authentic intimacy with your marriage partner.

At this point it's now easy! You've read through the Handbook—now highlight some of the practical ideas and action steps for:

- developing mental connections

- developing emotional connections

- developing spiritual connections, and

- developing sexual connections.

Practice them! Do them!

Take the time and effort to invest in your marriage by putting these tips, ideas, and suggestions into practice. We guarantee that your marriage will improve when you pursue your dream marriage through the loving actions and responses provided in these pages.

Contact Us

To book Jim and Carrie to speak at your church, event, or conference, or to reach them with any questions, contact them at:
contact@theintimatecouple.com
or reach out to them via social media:
facebook.com/intimate.couple.

Made in the USA
Columbia, SC
01 September 2024

40631891R00059